Paleo Diet

Paleo Diet Mistakes To Avoid For Rapid Weight Loss - The How To And Not To Guide For Beginners

Table of Contents

Not Making a Meal Plan

Not Keeping Tracks of Things.

Not Setting Milestones

Always Eating Out

Not Rewarding Yourself or Excessive Rewarding

The Solitary Reaper

Eating the Same Thing Everyday

No Exercise or Over-Exercise

No Sleep and Extreme Stress

Not Drinking Enough Water

Binge Eating

Unable to curb the Cravings

No Meat

Excessive Meat

Excessive Fruits

Excessive Nuts

Insufficient Vegetable intake

Wrong Condiments and Oils

Not Keeping a List of Things Allowed and Things Not
Allowed

Choosing the Wrong Paleo

Wrong Portion Sizes

Introduction

Due to rapid rise in industrialization and technological development, we are able to perform the most difficult, as well as highly trivial tasks with relative ease. Because of this, many of us lead an exceptionally sedentary life. However, human beings are not evolved to live a life without physical work, the absence of which has led to the rise of various diseases and disorders that plague the modern world. No wonder then, the fitness and health industry is growing at an exuberantly rapid scale nowadays.

Everyone you meet today is either trying to shed those extra pounds or is at least trying to maintain their body. As mentioned earlier, there has been a rapid and rather disturbing rise in the rate of obesity in people among all age groups. This has led to a market full of tall claims and false promises - claims that often harm more than heal.

It is all about speed and velocity today and people often try to find easier ways to drop off all the extra weight in a jiffy. One has to understand that the human body is not a machine, and cannot tolerate excess stress, thereby resulting in various problems. There are numerous fad diets that promise instant weight loss. What many people fail to grasp is that most of these diets are difficult to maintain and are highly unhealthy. Also, the results of these diets are often temporary and the effects wear off once you stop dieting. So, rather than focusing on such short-term diets, it is necessary to pick something that is well researched and scientifically proven.

There are a plethora of different kinds of diet plans that have been tested and scientifically proven. One such diet is the Paleo diet or the caveman diet that people are raving about. What makes Paleo diet effective for weight loss is that you are not left feeling hungry and exhausted, unlike many other diets. It is well researched, proven and effective. However, like every other diet you must avoid certain things and practices - mistakes that may ruin your complete routine.

This book will guide you through your Paleo diet weight loss plan and will help you to avoid some very common mistakes people make. You will also find basic information about Paleo diet, a specific meal plan, and answers to some frequently asked questions in this book as well. So, let's get started!

Chapter 1: Paleo Diet- Basics

What do you mean by Paleo diet? How does this diet work? Is it a fad diet? Is it trustworthy? Is it safe? How do I begin it?

Almost all of you have some, if not all the above questions in your minds right now. Don't worry; you are in the right place. This chapter will walk you through all the above queries and will serve as a total beginner's guide to the caveman's diet. For convenience, this chapter has been divided into various sub-chapters.

Paleo Diet- Introduction

You must have heard the term "Paleo diet" or "Paleo" quite often in health circles nowadays. It sounds like some new technical hogwash or one of those latest fad diets, isn't it? In fact, the reality is far from truth, because Paleo diet is really the oldest diet ever.

The diet or food that we consume nowadays is a highly recent phenomenon. Our dietary habits are only 10,000 years old. However, human beings have existed on this planet for more than two million years. Our recent diet is a mere fraction of the history of our dietary habits. What Paleo diet does is, it promotes you to consume food that was available 10,000 years ago. So, what did we eat 10,000 years ago?

It is a well-known fact that we started eating grains at a large scale and it became our staple only after the agricultural revolution. This revolution took about 10,000 years ago. Now that does not mean that we didn't eat grains before that, we did, but just the amount that was available naturally, without humans cultivating it. Basically, we ate everything edible that was available in the nature.

Our daily diet is full of sugar and processed foods, things that were not available to our ancestors. This includes grains too; and we all know that the human body doesn't digest grains easily. Turns out the human body has not evolved much through these years, and our bodies still are made to consume natural products.

The Paleo diet is therefore a diet that makes you go back in time, not a la 'Back to the Future' but in a gastronomic way. It is going back to eggs, meat, roots, nuts, fresh vegetables and fruits. You can basically eat everything that our ancestors may have eaten in the hunter/gatherer phase. So, no more cookies, cereals, pasta or any junk food that you would normally eat etc. No chemical, nothing processed and everything natural.

Some of the most common Paleo foods include natural oils such as coconut oil, olive oil, various nuts and roots, fish, seafood, vegetables, eggs and fruits. Lean meats too form an integral part of the Paleo diet.

All these changes in your daily diet can lead to innumerable benefits, easing your way through the weight loss journey. Let's have a look at some of the major advantages of this diet in the next section.

Benefits of Paleo Diet

Easy Weight Loss

Let's start with the benefit that most of the people seek when they start a dieting regime- weight loss. What makes Paleo diet particularly effective in this field is that you will start losing weight within no time. As you are only supposed to eat natural foods while on a Paleo diet, it leads to decreased consumption of unnatural and processed foods. What makes Paleo diet easy to follow and an effortless way to lose weight is that you don't have to stop eating or measure calories all the time.

Unlike other diets where you have to watch every calorie that you consume and starve yourself, Paleo diet gives you a free reign to eat whatever you want (albeit only the things that are allowed on the diet). This freedom makes the rather cumbersome process of going on a diet quite easy and doable. You will start to enjoy the process after sometime and will forget that you are on a diet, all the while losing weight continuously! Due to the fun factor of the diet you won't feel miserable at all. This in turn allows you to stick to the regime and avoid resentment.

Detox

You must have heard people going on detox diets all the time. Detox diets plans have become so important in today's world, thanks to the ever-increasing pollution and impurities in the environment. These impurities travel and settle in our body due to ecological carriers and food. Some of the most harmful toxins settle in our body when we consume large amounts of trans-fats, foods full of MSG, refined sugar, caffeine etc. However, as Paleo diet involves eating only natural foods you automatically bypass these harmful additives giving your body a much-needed rest.

Paleo diet promotes a healthy diet by consuming natural foods, which help you to detoxify your body. Natural foods are rich sources of fiber, antioxidants and phytonutrients. These nutrients are essential in purgation of the accumulated toxins from the body, leaving the body feeling lighter and much more active. The benefit of Paleo for detox is that unlike other detox routines you don't have to go on a fluid only diet while trying hard to curb your cravings. Instead, you can reap almost similar benefits while eating regular meals.

Cutting off Junk Food and Fast Food

The pressures of this fast paced world also affect our dietary habits. More and more people are relying solely upon junk food to satisfy their hunger. It is a well-known fact that excessive junk food or fast food is extremely harmful for your health. Junk food contains almost zero essential nutrients and pack hefty amounts of processed foods and ingredients. Often these processed foods are full of synthetic chemicals. While on Paleo, you are supposed to steer off junk food thus saving your body from high cholesterol and other harmful disorders. You will also start saving a lot of money that you normally spend on junk food. This money can be spent on organic foods that will help you in your Paleo diet regime.

Cutting down on junk food from your diet might prove to be a gruesome task for many in the beginning. It is not only a psychological adjustment, but physical as well, which shows how much these foods have ensnared our diets. For instance, several brands of milk cookies are almost as addictive as morphine or cocaine. They activate the pleasure centers of the brain even better than various drugs. This is also true in the case of potato chips and French fries. However, with little dedication and effort you will be able to overcome these substances with ease.

Better Sleeping Patterns

One of the most essential activities for every living being is sleep. We may not know everything about sleep patterns, but we do know that it is highly essential and that uncomfortable sleeping patterns may ruin your life. Processed foods often contain chemicals such as caffeine and various others, which interfere with the natural sleeping pattern that result into bad sleep.

Often serotonin, the natural compound that brain releases to make you sleepy gets overridden by all the additives from processed foods. However, on Paleo diet you will consume only natural foods that will help you to sleep better. Not only will you sleep well but you will also rise bright and feeling energized after a few days of Paleo diet. This is a sign of your body tuning itself per the natural circadian cycle, just like our ancestors.

Prevent Diseases and Disorders

As stated earlier processed foods are one of the major culprits in the rise of obesity and diabetes all over the world. These foods contain various harmful compounds as well as fillers that serve no purpose other than taste. Some of the chemicals present in various processed foodstuffs are so harmful that they may lead to disorders such as cancer, cardiac problems, hepatic problems, pancreatic diseases, diabetes etc.

Many processed foods also contain large amounts of preservatives. Chemicals such BHA or butylated hydroxyanisole and BHT or butylated hydroxytoluene have been proved to affect your neurological system, and are also known to cause cancer. On a Paleo diet, you can avoid all the harmful chemicals without any additional labor. As mentioned above Paleo food contains high number of phytonutrients and antioxidants that not only keep you energized but can also fight against the above-mentioned diseases to a certain extent.

No Cumbersome Calorie Counting

One of the most cumbersome and tedious tasks related to dieting is the strict measurement and accounting of calories consumed and burned. In almost all diets, you are made to keep a close eye on what are you eating and how much you are eating. You are often made to carry calorie charts and calorie calculators so that you do not consume more than the stipulated amount. But this is all old school; in Paleo diet you are never haunted by numbers, as you never count calories. It is easy to follow and intrinsically simple. There are no hard and fixed rules for Paleo diet and you do not have limit yourself.

Satiation

For most of the people diet equals to constant hunger, and it is true in the case of most of the diets. However, in Paleo diet you never feel hungry or go to sleep with an empty stomach. Paleo diet consists of high amounts of fiber and healthy fats that keep you feeling full for a long time. You can often go without cravings for days. If you eat right amounts of veggies, fruits and meat in every meal you can easily work throughout the day without feeling hungry at all.

Maintains Healthy Blood Glucose Levels

Unknowingly, we consume way more sugar every day than we are supposed to. Almost every other food item we eat is full of sugar. Excess sugar makes the blood Glucose levels shoot up drastically and makes it fluctuate more often. However, as start cutting off every food item with added processed sugar while on Paleo diet, you effectively help your body to maintain the blood glucose levels. You won't feel fatigued because of frequent sugar crashes either. If you were trying to avoid diabetes, then this diet would be your best bet. However, if you are already a diabetic it is advised that you consult your physician before beginning this diet.

Gluten Free

In the recent few years there has been an epidemical rise in the popularity of gluten free food items. Almost everyone who keeps up with the times has heard of gluten free diets that help the body stay fit and active. Paleo diet too is a gluten free diet as you avoid almost all grains while following it.

Many studies have emerged stating that gluten often interferes with digestion and assimilation, and often results in IBS as well as rapid weight gain. This is also true in the case of people who do not suffer from Celiac disease or gluten sensitivity. By cutting off gluten from your diet, you can keep your gut healthy which in turn will reduce the sedateness associated with indigestion.

Healthy Body Cells and Healthy Brian

Human body is made of innumerable cells and these cells are made of saturated and unsaturated fats. The health of the cell is solely dependent upon the perfect balance between the two fats. Paleo diet is one of the few diets that help your body to maintain this balance effectively as you are supposed to eat both kinds of fats while following the diet. This is different than many other diets where only one kind of fats are preferred.

Paleo diet is beneficial for the brain and nervous system as well. Salmon is a highly recommended food item for everyone who wants to follow the Paleo diet. Salmon is full of omega 3 fatty acids, which are often lacking in an average American person. Omega 3 contains high amounts of DHA, a compound that is essential for the health of eyes, brain and the heart. Omega 3 is also present in pasture grown eggs and meat.

Reducing Allergies and Inflammation

Many food items contain allergens that can prove to be harmful for a large chunk of the population. Two of the most common allergy causing foot items are grains and milk both of which are to be avoided on a Paleo diet. Milk is often a controversial topic for Paleo followers but more on it later. Paleo diet is also full of anti-inflammatory food items such as various herbs and veggies that help you to avoid the inflammation of heart, stomach etc.

Cutting off Empty Calories

Do you know you can lose a considerable amount of weight just by avoiding sodas and beers? Beverages such as sodas, beers and many other sugary drinks are full of what are known, as empty calories i.e. they serve no nutritional purpose however are full of calories. These drinks are often full of sugar and chemicals.

Paleo diet makes you automatically avoid these drinks and thus in turn avoid the chemicals and sugar as well. Some of you may ask what to do when you need an extra surge of energy and are not allowed to drink energy drinks? Paleo diet can successfully curb such cravings too.

Energizing Foodstuffs

Paleo diet is full of naturally produced vegetables, fruits, roots etc. When combined properly a Paleo meal has right and balanced proportions of proteins, minerals, vitamins, carbs and all nutrients. This nutrient rich food will keep you energized throughout the day without the lethargic side effects of sugary drinks.

Easy to Follow

Paleo recipes are extremely easy and do not take a lot of time to prepare. Almost all ingredients are fresh which reduces the cooking time quite significantly. You don't have worry about calorie counts and proportions while cooking Paleo meals. On the contrary, you can eat everything that is allowed on a Paleo diet at every meal.

In this chapter, we saw a basic introduction of Paleo diet and went through the numerous benefits of the diet. These benefits must have got you even more curious about the diet, but some of you might be wondering how does a simple diet like this work so well for us. In the next chapter we are going to have close look at how effective Paleo diet is.

Chapter 2: The Workings of Paleo Diet

How does Paleo diet work?

Before looking at how Paleo diet works let's throw some light about an important fact. When someone talks about our ancestors from 10,000 years ago, most of you would imagine a tall, dark, lean, agile and muscular person ready to do anything to sustain. Now imagine a modern-day human being. We immediately picture a fat, lazy, sedentary, stressed out and out of shape individual who is also extremely unhappy, and probably has some sort of chronic disorder. So, what happened in just 10,000 years that changed us so much?

The answer is discovery of agriculture. Now it is impossible to imagine a world without agriculture as everything that we see around us today. Every form of material as well as spiritual progress has evolved from the development of agriculture, but it undoubtedly ruined our dietary habits as well.

Before the discovery of agriculture, almost every human was either a gatherer or a hunter- they used to gather fruits, roots, and vegetables or hunt animals/ fish or in many cases both. The human body, especially the digestive system, was developed for this kind of diet full of natural products. It took us millions of years to develop a strong digestive system that supported this kind of diet. However, after the discovery of agriculture, we settled down and stopped hunting and gathering.

Grains became our staple diet while the other dietary forms took lesser positions. What is remarkable is that the human body and human digestive system is still in the pre-agriculture mode i.e. our body is still most suitable for products of the hunting/ gathering mode of production. This digestive system is not made for processing grains and lags.

Seasonal vegetables and fruits, lean meats, fish etc. are supposed to form a major portion our diet, which unfortunately has been replaced by grains and large amounts of processed foods such as pasta, bread, rice etc. This overloading of grains along with increasingly sedentary lifestyle leads to obesity and many diseases and disorders

Paleo is all about going back to our roots and eating like our forefathers did, for we are closely connected to them. Moving on towards the effectiveness of Paleo diet we find that Paleo diet is effective way to turn your body into a weight loss machine. It achieves this goal as follows.

Human body loves fats. Almost everything we consume gets stored in the body as fats (if not used soon). For instance, if you consume wheat it is broken down in the body to release the carbohydrates. These carbohydrates are turned into glucose by the body. Glucose is a type of sugar that provides us with energy to do various tasks. However, if we fail to burn off this glucose in a stipulated time our body starts converting and storing it as fats.

In today's world, we often consume a lot of carbohydrates. Our body burns them for our day-to-day energy. However due to the imbalanced ratio of the carbs consumed and energy used, our body often stores excessive converted fats in our cells. This process is one of the remnants of the past days when humans were solely dependent on hunting and gathering for food and often had to go without it for days. However, in modern world many of us are privileged enough to get more than our needs that result into a never-ending stack of fats.

Paleo diet forces you to remove most of the carbohydrates from your diet. This lack of carbohydrates forces your body to burn the stored fats instead to provide itself with energy. Without the continuous bombardment of carbs, the body also does not produce extra sugar. This very thing in turn helps you to regulate your insulin levels. This stage is known as ketosis in scientific terms, and Paleo being one of the many ketogenic diets.

In the next chapter, we are going to learn all about how to begin a Paleo diet.

Chapter 3: A Basic Guideline for Paleo Diet

In this chapter, you will find a detailed guideline that will help any beginner to start Paleo diet. You will find out what are you supposed to do before you begin the Paleo diet including things that will keep you motivated through it.

Hunting and Gathering food

Unlike our ancestors, you don't have to hunt animals and gather fruits for the diet. Instead you can hunt and throw away all the food items that are not allowed on a Paleo diet from your pantry. Along with the hunting, gather all the items that you find necessary for your Paleo diet meal plan. You can find an extensive shopping list in next chapter that will help you choose wisely. You will also find a 'What to Avoid' list in latter chapter that will help you to steer off harmful products. Cleaning your pantry should be your priority, as this will make it easy to avoid temptations.

If you are not comfortable with throwing away and dropping your favorite foods all at once you can do them week by week, i.e. you can throw away the dairy in the first week followed by grains the next. Keep doing this until you get onto your Paleo diet. While stocking your pantry with Paleo food you can also invest in good cookware. Many Paleo recipes are prepared in a crockpot and if you don't have one buy as soon as possible. Crockpot will make cooking and in turn your life much easier.

Remember to keep your pantry stocked with Paleo friendly food on your day offs from work.

Develop a Meal Plan

Every individual is different and hence their bodily requirements as well as their motives behind doing the diet are different. Formulate a diet/meal plan that fulfills all your needs and requirements. You can chalk out all the recipes that you want to make throughout the month making the diet highly convenient. It also makes shopping highly convenient. You'll find a sample two-week plan in the next chapter.

Stay Motivated

Each day thousands of people go on various kinds of diets but at the end of the week only few hundred remain true to their plans. Why do most of them fall off their plans? A very simple answer to this question is lack of motivation. Human beings need some sort of motivation to perform any task and when the amount of motivation is not proportional to the magnitude of the task, we fail.

Dieting sounds simple but is often a brutal task. Many people fail to curb cravings and indulge in binge eating. To avoid this, concentrate on your goals, for instance if weight loss is your goal then focus only on losing weight. Subscribe to various motivational quotes sites and try out some motivational audio playlists. Set reminders on your smartphone to remind and motivate you to continue your diet. You can also ask your friends and family to help you achieve your goals.

Scale and Tape

One of the most necessary things to keep you motivated is to track your progress. It takes weeks before you start noticing weight loss with your naked eyes, however a weighing scale and measuring tape will see the difference as soon as it starts. These little achievements can keep you motivated and can help you track your diet as well. However, don't go obsessing over it.

Modification

When eating out with friends or going for a business dinner you can still follow Paleo diet. It is all about how well you can read the menu. Choose the dishes that are the most Paleo friendly. For instance, if you order salmon and veggies, you can request the restaurant to avoid condiments such as soy sauce and perhaps replace rice with double veggies.

Learn Cooking

This might seem a bit daunting to people who have never cooked anything in their life. However, while on the Paleo diet you will often need to eat things that people normally don't. Almost everyone eats grains and dairy every day, hence you will need separate foods. It is almost impossible to control the ingredients used in a restaurant as well as when somebody cooks for you. You can feel free to experiment with recipes and food items to create your own, tasty dishes. You can also try the numerous Paleo recipe books that are available online. Most of the Paleo recipes are easy to make/bake, which even a beginner can emulate with ease.

Understand Labels

Although you are not supposed to keep a close eye on the number of calories it is necessary to read labels of products before you buy them. Many food items that appear innocent can throw off your Paleo diet. For instance, condiments, such as soy sauce, many marinades, sauces etc. and peanut butter are NOT Paleo. Read the ingredients of the products before adding them to your shopping cart.

Now let's look at the basic meal plan that an adult can follow on a Paleo diet. A short list of Paleo foodstuffs will be provided along with the plan in the next chapter so that you can chalk out your own plan effectively.

Chapter 4: Simple Paleo Diet Meal Plan and List of Necessary Food Items

Paleo diet is one of the few revolutionary diets available for human kind because you don't have to count calories in your food and keep an eye on every nutritional index; you are free to eat whatever you want to. However, for better results it is necessary to sketch a plan and follow it, but don't worry the plan given in this chapter is nowhere a concrete plan. You can modify it per your requirements and can form your own Paleo diet meal plan easily. Before moving on to the meal plan let us have a look at some of the most common food items that are allowed on a Paleo diet.

Paleo Foods/ Shopping List

Here you will find a comprehensive and well-sorted list of food products that you may choose and buy per your tastes and needs. You don't have to buy every item from the list however it is advised that you do stock at least two items from each category.

Meat

Some people call Paleo diet a meat heavy diet and it is true. Although many vegetarian iterations of the diet exist, common diet plans still are heavily focused on meats. Almost all meats are, in a way, Paleo meats. However, what makes Paleo meats different from other meats is how much they have been processed. Sausages, spam etc. should be avoided on Paleo diet. It is highly recommended that you buy grass fed meat instead of grain fed meat while on Paleo diet. As this diet is based on the ancient hunters you can also try exotic meat (legally procured).

- Turkey

- Poultry

- Veal

- Chicken (breasts)

- Pork Chops

- Pork Tenderloin

- Bacon

- Steak

- Beef (ground)

- Pork

- Chicken (thigh)

- Chicken (wings)

- Chicken (leg)

- Lamb

PALEO DIET

- Venison
- Bison (jerky)
- Bison (steaks)
- Bison (sirloin)
- Bison (ribs)
- Lamb (chops)
- Elk
- Rabbit
- Buffalo
- Goat
- Emu
- Kangaroo
- Goose
- Duck
- Wild Boar
- Ostrich
- Quail
- Turtle
- Rattle Snake

- Pheasant

- Deer

Organs Such As

- Livers

- Kidneys

- Foot

- Heart

- Marrow

- Tongue

- Sweetbreads

Vegetables

Almost all vegetables are Paleo, or they were, once upon a time. Owing to the use of excessive chemicals and hybridization, our vegetables look and taste considerably different than those that were available to our ancestors. However, you can still consume almost all organically grown vegetables while following a Paleo diet. Just eat potatoes and squashes in moderation and you are good to go.

- Avocado

- Celery

- Asparagus

- Spinach
- Potato
- Carrots
- Brussels Sprouts
- Broccoli
- Butternut Squash
- Artichoke
- Sweet Potato
- Zucchini
- Yam
- Peppers (all types)
- Onions
- Cauliflower
- Beetroot
- Green Onion
- Parsley
- Cabbage
- Eggplant

Fruits

After vegetables, fruits are an essential part of a Paleo diet as well. They are tasty and are good for your skin, hair and overall health. However, certain fruits contain high amounts of natural sugar as well. If you are aiming for weight loss you, should eat such fruits in moderation. Remember, our ancestors didn't have abundance of fruits and nuts available.

- Avocado

- Grapes

- Apple

- Blackberries

- Plums

- Blueberries

- Papaya

- Peaches

- Lychee

- Lemon

- Mango

- Watermelon

- Lime

- Figs

- Oranges

- Banana

- Strawberries

- Guava

- Raspberries

- Tangerines

- Cantaloupe

Sea Food

Paleo diet is based on the diet of ancient hunters and gatherers and fishing involves both the elements. Seafoods contain high amounts of omega 3 compounds that are essential for human body. Let us have a look at some of the seafood that you can eat while on a Paleo diet.

- Salmon (must eat this)

- Anchovies

- Clams

- Bass

- Crayfish

- Halibut

- Sardines

- Shellfish Tuna

PALEO DIET

- Cod
- Crab
- Red Snapper
- Lobster
- Mackerel
- Flounder
- Shrimp
- Tuna
- Scallops
- Sunfish
- Mussels
- Shark
- Mahi Mahi
- Crawfish
- Swordfish
- Trout
- Tilapia
- Oysters
- Walleye

Oils and Nuts

You must be wondering what this section is doing in a diet book. But that is the benefit of Paleo diet. You are encouraged to consume moderate amounts of healthy fats on this diet to keep you active and fit. Nuts are rich sources of good fats and therefore should be consumed in moderation while on Paleo diet. Try to avoid fried and processed nuts.

Oils

- Macadamia Oil
- Coconut Oil
- Almond Oil
- Flaxseed Oil
- Walnut Oil
- Avocado Oil
- Olive Oil
- Butter (grass fed)

Nuts and Seeds

- Cashews
- Pecans
- Sesame Seeds

- Macadamia Nuts

- Almonds

- Pistachio

- Pine Nuts

- Hazelnuts

- Flax Seeds

- Brazil Nuts

- Pumpkin Seeds

- Walnuts

- Sunflower Seeds

Beverages

- Water

- Lemon water

- Fruit Infused Water

- Coconut water

- Coconut milk

- Soda water

Treats

- Paleo Friendly Muffins/ desserts

- Raw Honey

- Coconut products

- Maple Syrup

Meal Plan

Here, we have provided a simple two-week meal plan for people who want to lose weight. It is a generic plan that you can modify per your needs and body. If you are an athlete or are more sedentary than others, check the "How to" chapter to modulate the diet plan.

Week 1

Monday

Breakfast

- Baked Chicken

Lunch

- Chicken Salad

Dinner

- Rogan Josh

Side Dish (Lunch or Dinner)

- Steamed Cabbage

Snack

- Handful of nuts

Desserts

- Watermelon slices

Tuesday

Breakfast

- Eggs with Bacon and onion

Lunch

- Beef Brisket with Mushrooms

Dinner

- Chicken and Kale with desired vegetable dressing

Side Dish

- Chopped Cucumber and Radishes with Olive Oil

Snack

- Baked Jalapenos stuffed with cucumber

Dessert

- Baked Apple Slices

Wednesday

Breakfast

- Steamed Veggies

Lunch

- Pan fried Salmon with onions

Dinner

- Grain less Pizza

Side Dish

- Baked Broccoli with roasted prosciutto and chili vinegar

Snack

- Crispy Nuts

Dessert

- Gingerbread Cookies

Thursday

Breakfast

- Sweet Potato Hash with ground beef and pepper

Lunch

- Africa style Chicken

Dinner

- Pot roast with tomatoes

Side Dish

- Baked Brussels sprouts

Snack

- Yogurt Nuts

Dessert

- Fruit Salad

Friday

Breakfast

- Lightly toasted Kale with Bacon

Lunch

- Pan Fried Bass with an Egg

Dinner

- Chicken Salad in Moroccan Style

Side Dish

- Celery Salad with cherry tomatoes

Snack

- Carrot sticks with cabbage mush

Dessert

- Baked Apple and Peach slices

Saturday

Breakfast

- Light Casserole

Lunch

- Chicken Fajita Salad

Dinner

- Rogan Josh

Side Dish

- Steamed Carrots with Red wine

Snack

- Cucumber slices with pesto

Dessert

- Small mango

Sunday

Breakfast

- Batter less Pancakes with berries

Lunch

- Salmon Cakes

Dinner

- Lamb Chops

Side Dish

- Green salad with balsamic vinegar

Snack

- Apple

Dessert

- Roasted Coconut with Kiwi

Week 2

Monday

Breakfast

- Veggie Cakes and cottage cheese

Lunch

- Pork Chops

Dinner

- Pot Roast

Side Dish

- Steamed Cauliflower

Snack

- Baba Ganoush

Dessert

- Yogurt and coconut

Tuesday

Breakfast

- Baked Cauliflowers

Lunch

- Roasted Mushrooms with bell pepper

Dinner

- Lamb Roast with beet sauce

Side Dish

- Kale Salad with sesame

Snack

- Almond Salad with cilantro

Dessert

- Small banana with cashews

Wednesday

Breakfast

- Curried Potatoes

Lunch

- Chicken Salad in Moroccan Style

Dinner

- Pan Fried Bass with an Egg
- *Side Dish*

Meatloaves

Snack

- Roasted button mushrooms with black pepper

Dessert

- Almonds

Thursday

Breakfast

- Stir fried zucchini with scrambled eggs

Lunch

- Baked Salmon in onion and tomato gravy

Dinner

- Moroccan Chicken Salad

Side Dish

- Green Salad with White Wine

Snack

- Soft Boiled eggs with roasted bell pepper

Dessert

- Coconut milk with Walnut

Friday

Breakfast

- Sautéed Kale and Cherry tomatoes

Lunch

- Baked Butternut squash

Dinner

- Carrots and beet in ginger garlic with tomato sauce

Side Dish

- Celery Salad with cherry tomatoes

Snack

- Crispy Nuts

Dessert

- Mango with sticky rice

Saturday

Breakfast

- Bratwurst with German Salad

Lunch

- Chicken Fajita Salad

Dinner

- Tomato curry with Eggplant

Side Dish

- Greens and Roasted Mushroom

Snack

- Beef Jerky

Dessert

- Coconut Milk Ice Cream

Sunday

Breakfast

- Scrambled eggs with roasted bell peppers

Lunch

- Easy Roast Chicken

Dinner

- Pumpkin Curry

Side Dish

- Stuffed Mushrooms

Snack

- Salmon Stuffed Avocado

Dessert

- Pecan Sandies

Along with the meal plan, we have included a few recipes that you can try before starting the diet to understand how tasty Paleo food can be.

Paleo Diet Recipes

1. Pan Fried Liver with Bacon and Onions
Ingredients

- 1-2-piece bacon

- 1 onion, large, chopped

- 1 small liver (turkey or chicken)

- 1 tbsp. coconut oil

- 12-15 almonds

- Paprika or crushed black pepper per taste

- ¼ tsp. nutmeg powder

- Salt per taste

- 2 tbsps. Ghee

- 2 tbsps. Lightly chopped cilantro

Instructions

1. Roast bacon lightly in a frying pan on medium heat. Keep aside when done.

2. In another pan stir fry onion slices in 1 tbsp. coconut oil over medium heat. Add salt and pepper per taste. Sauté for 10-15 minutes or till the onions get caramelized fully. Keep aside.

3. Pulse almonds until a flour like consistency is achieved. You can also use pre-made almond flour.

4. In a bowl add the almond flour, paprika or pepper, salt and nutmeg. Mix well.

5. Rinse and pat dry the liver and make about ½ inch slices.

6. In another pan heat ghee.

7. Dredge the liver slices in the almond flour carefully. Make sure to coat it well.

8. Stir-fry the liver slices in ghee for about two minutes on each side.

9. To serve place the hot liver slices on a dish and top them with the onions. Put the bacon slices over the onions and garnish with cilantro or parsley.

2. Cucumber and dried fish Salad
Ingredients

- ¾ cups dried fish

- 3 medium cucumbers, chopped thinly

- 5 tbsps. Olive oil (sesame oil can be used as well)

- 2 tbsps. Apple cider vinegar (lime juice can be used as well)

- Salt to taste

- Sesame seeds for garnish

Instructions

1. Take a large mixing bowl and add all the ingredients one by one.

2. Toss well.

3. While serving add more dressing if needed.

3. Coconut Macaroons
Ingredients

- ½ cup walnuts, soaked

- 1 small cup dates, seeded and roughly chopped

- Vanilla Extract

- ½ tsp ginger, chopped

- 2 cups coconut flakes

- 2 tbsps. Coconut cream

- Coconut oil for greasing

Instructions

1. Keep the oven on preheat mode at 350 F for 10 minutes.

2. In a mixing bowl add walnuts, ginger, vanilla extract

and ginger and mix well. Pulse this mixture in a food processor. Remove and keep aside.

3. Add coconut cream and coconut flakes to the food processor and pulse. Now add the above mixture to the food processor and pulse till all the ingredients are combined. Remove in a bowl.

4. Knead the mixture with your hands and keep aside.

5. Take a baking dish and grease it lightly with the coconut oil. Grease your palms lightly as well.

6. Make small cookie sized balls and flatten them on the baking dish. Remember these will not change shape after baking!

7. Bake for 25-30 minutes at 350 F.

4. Paleo Breakfast Sausage
Ingredients

- 3 lbs. pork, ground

- 3 tsp. sage, lightly crushed

- 3-5 cloves garlic, lightly crushed

- 4 green onions, chopped roughly

- 1 1/2 tbsp maple syrup

- 1 1/2 tbsp lemon juice

- Salt to taste

- Pepper, freshly ground

- Cayenne, to taste

- Red chili flakes

Instructions

1. Take a large mixing bowl and add all the ingredients one by one while keeping the pork aside. Mix everything well until combined properly.

2. Add pork to the above mixture and mix well.

3. Grease your palms lightly with any Paleo friendly oil and make small patties of the pork mixture.

4. Heat a large frying pan on medium heat and brown the patties on both the sides.

5. Serve hot with your favorite dip.

5. Indian Style Paleo Chicken Stew
Ingredients

- 2 tbsp coconut oil, divided

- 2 chicken breasts, boneless

- Salt, to taste

- Ground pepper, fresh

- 1 yellow onion, chopped

- 1 inch piece of ginger, minced

- 4-6 cloves garlic, minced

- 1 1/4 tbsp garam masala

- Cayenne, to taste

- 1 1/2 tsp cumin

- 1/2 tsp coriander powder

- 2 1/2 cups homemade chicken broth

- 1/4 cup coconut cream

- 1 cup tomato puree

- 2 sweet potatoes, small, peeled and diced

- Cilantro, for garnish

Instructions

1. Marinate chicken for 10 minutes by coating it with generous amount of salt and pepper.

2. Take a Dutch oven and heat 1 tbsp coconut oil in it on medium. Place the chicken in the oven and let it brown in each side for five minutes. Generously season the

chicken with salt and pepper and place into the pan. Brown on each side for 4-5 minutes. Remove and keep aside.

3. In the same oven add the rest of the oil and heat it on medium heat again. When hot enough add garlic, onions and ginger. Sauté for 5-8 minutes till the onions become translucent.

4. Once onions become soft enough, add cumin, garam masala, coriander and cayenne along with one tbsp of tomato puree. Mix well and let it simmer for 4-5 minutes.

5. Add broth, chicken breasts and all the remaining puree to the pot. Let it boil and. then reduce the heat. Let it cook with a lid on for about 1 1/2 hours on low to medium heat.

6. Take off the lid after 1 1/2 hours season the stew with salt and pepper. Take out all the chicken pieces and shred them lightly. Re-add the chicken along with the sweet potato to the pot and let cook for around 30-40 minutes with lid closed. Stir occasionally.

7. Add coconut milk during the last 4-5 minutes turn off the heat.

8. Garnish with cilantro.

Chapter 5: Mistakes to Avoid on a Paleo Diet

Diet followers often come across setbacks that sometimes throw them off routine. This is perfectly natural and happens with almost everyone. However, instead of dwelling upon it, it is necessary to pick yourself and stick to the diet. In this chapter, you will find common mistakes that trouble every Paleo follower and tips and tricks that will solve these problems. You will learn what to do and what to avoid while following a Paleo diet.

Not Making a Meal Plan

Not having a meal plan is one of the most common mistakes that beginners make while beginning a Paleo diet. By making meal plans you can avoid accidental binge eating and can keep a track of your diet. You will make fewer mistakes than on an unplanned diet.

It is also necessary to modify your diet plan per your bodily needs. For instance, athletes should eat a protein rich diet supplemented by enough carbs while people who are trying to lose weight should avoid carbs as much as possible and need to consume moderate amount of fats.

Not Keeping Tracks of Things.

The best motivation you can find is to keep a track of your progress. Keeping a track of things in a journal will not only help you to notice your achievements, but you will also be able to improvise your weight loss plans. Make regular entries in your journals so that you can gauge whether you are going in the right direction, and can modify your routine accordingly. However, if you avoid keeping a journal you won't be able to mark your progress and your diet may suddenly go downhill if it hits a rough spot.

If you find journaling boring or cumbersome, you can try the various apps that are available for almost all smartphones. These apps are easy to use and can be carried around all over. Other than apps, you can write blogs about your diet routine that will not only help you to keep a track of your plan, but will also help the others looking for motivation.

Not Setting Milestones

You have seen it; you have perhaps experienced it. All of us choose a diet and set a goal only to fail after few days. This happens because more than often a lot of people choose huge and daunting goals. Instead of picking up an extensive and gigantic goal, try and divide it into smaller ones. For instance, if you want to lose 20 pounds, instead of making a huge plan to lose them all together make smaller plans. For instance, you can start with 5 pounds and gradually increase the target. This will keep you motivated, as you will continuously get a feeling of achievement. Remember a smaller goal is easily doable.

Always Eating Out

Due to our hectic and always on toes life it is impossible to avoid eating out. However, as most restaurants are not Paleo friendly, your diet can go on a toss. While following Paleo diet, try and avoid eating out as much as possible. This includes dinners with friends, dates, parties, and eating at the office as well. However, you don't have to kill your social life to lose weight. Carry your food with you to the places where you can get away with it. Throw some house parties, which will enable you to keep a close eye on the food and drinks. It is also possible to go out and do activities that do not concern food and drinks or choose wisely so that you can eat out and still stay true to your diet.

Not Rewarding Yourself or Excessive Rewarding

We love rewards and although the weight loss and other health benefits are significant rewards themselves, for some people they are not enough to keep them on track. Reward yourself time to time with various activities and sometimes non-Paleo snacks to keep your brain happy. If you divide your diet plan into small parts, you can have a reward at the end of each part. Rewards may include a trip to spa, a small chocolate bar etc. Remember, these little rewards can go long way and can make the whole process fun and interesting.

Although rewards are essential, they are to be had in moderation. One tiny mistake and your plans may fall flat. Portioning/rationing of food related rewards are necessary. In the case of other forms of rewards, it is necessary keep yourself from going overboard and spending a lot of money. Remember, you are doing this diet for weight loss and not as an excuse to buy things.

The Solitary Reaper

Human beings love competition. Almost all of us perform our best when we have someone to compete with and when we have people supporting us. Ask a friend to be your diet partner. This way you can stay on your routine for a longer time. You can keep an eye on each other's diet, which will help you to adhere to it strictly.

You can also join various offline and online support groups. It is not necessary to find a Paleo specific group; any diet group can prove to be helpful. In a diet group, you would be able to hear and share your journey. You can also get free advice to increase the effect of your diet. If you don't want to join an online group and cannot find a real one around you, invest some time and consider starting one yourself.

Although Paleo diet is a rapid weight loss diet, it is not a quick and superfast method to lose weight. You simply cannot expect to fit in your old jeans just after a week of Paleo. Paleo diet is a well-researched diet plan that helps you lose weight along with other things in a healthy manner. Diets and exercise routines that promise instant weight loss or muscle gains are either fake or are extremely unhealthy.

It takes time and dedication to follow a Paleo lifestyle. Many Paleo followers often complain of bloating, fatigue and feeling starved in the first week or two of Paleo diet. However, there's no reason to worry and do not stop, this is perfectly natural. Your body is going through a transitional period and it will take time to adjust. However, if the feeling of starvation does not go away in a couple of weeks increase your portion size, you are probably under eating.

In the later and early stages of the diet you may get what is called as 'carb flu'. Symptoms of this flu

Eating the Same Thing Everyday

Change is the ultimate truth of life and variety its essence. Experiment with your recipes and try not to repeat them more than once a week. A monotonous diet plan will make the dieting experience quite unhappy and difficult to follow. Buy some good Paleo recipe books if you are afraid to experiment. Alternating recipes will also help you to get the required nutrients without taking additional supplements.

No Exercise or Over-Exercise

Any diet, even a great one like Paleo will not help you to lose weight rapidly unless you accompany it with a good exercise plan. It is necessary to exercise at least thrice a week. You cannot experience the full benefits of a Paleo diet unless you undertake some sort of physical activity. However, it is not necessary to join a gym for this. A 30 minutes walk everyday can prove to be quite beneficial. If you wish to add some excitement, take up a sport like tennis, racquetball etc. You can also try swimming. Remember it is all about being active.

Whatever exercise routine you undertake, please remember to coordinate it with your diet. It is necessary to eat per you exercise routine to keep your body healthy. Excessive exercise combined with Paleo may cause harm, as you do not get the required carbs for strenuous workout. Instead of hardcore workout routine pick up lighter things such as Zumba, Yoga or cardio routines. These go perfectly well with a Paleo lifestyle and will leave you feeling refreshed.

No Sleep and Extreme Stress

Dieting can be a daunting experience that can be stressful for many. It is necessary to relax and calm down. Beat out stress by taking up activities such as reading or keeping yourself entertained with music and movies. You can also take up yoga and meditation to keep stress at bay. Avoid addicting substances such as alcohol and smoking. Remember, Paleo diet is a detox diet that clears out impurities from the body, so avoid adding them again.

Sleep is extremely essential for the overall well being of the body as well as for weight loss. It is necessary to get a good night's sleep for at least six hours. Avoid using mobile phones, tablets etc. right before you sleep, these emit blue light that is harmful for your circadian rhythm.

Not Drinking Enough Water

Dieting is not all about food, water forms an essential part of it as well. As Paleo diet is a fiber rich diet it becomes necessary to consume at least 10-12 glasses of water every day to prevent constipation and bloating. Water also satiates you, which prevents over eating. If you don't like to drink plain water invest in a good infuser and drink fruit water. You can also drink lemon water, orange juice etc. However, do not drink packaged juices as they contain high amounts of sugar and chemicals.

If you find it difficult to remember to drink water you can download various reminder apps available for almost all smartphones. These are specifically developed to remind you to drink water time to time.

If you do feel bloated occasionally, just drink plenty of water and try some home remedies.

Binge Eating

Stress and tension often results into binge eating. Everyone loves to eat chips and popcorn while watching a movie or a TV show. However, this can throw you off diet. Instead pick up things like cucumber, celery etc. to binge eat. These food items contain low calories and are Paleo friendly. They also contain various nutrients and are not empty calories like chips.

Unable to curb the Cravings

Cravings are inevitable. You will feel a strong craving for something or the other occasionally. Cravings for sugar are one of the most common cravings. However, instead of succumbing to the cravings, try to bypass them with a few smart moves. If you feel like eating something sweet such as a cookie or muffin eat some fruit instead. Many Paleo followers swear upon mango to curb the cravings. However, eat these treats in moderation. After sometime your body will get accustomed to the diet and you will find cookies and muffins to be too sweet to your taste.

You can often find "Paleo" marked upon a lot of products that are not traditionally Paleo. For instance, it is easy to find Paleo bread, Paleo muffins, Paleo ice cream etc. in a supermarket. You can also find thousands of Paleo friendly recipes for cakes, ice creams and all forms of desserts. However, these goods can ruin your diet. Just because mangoes are Paleo friendly doesn't mean that you can eat dozens of them together.

The items mentioned above are 100% Paleo items but still are unhealthy. For instance, a Paleo muffin may not contain grains and gluten but it is still full of sugar and lacks other nutrients such as proteins, vitamins etc. Using these to satisfy your cravings will not help you at all. Remember your digestive system does not understand the source of sugar and treats all forms of it in a similar manner.

That said you may eat such items sparingly often as rewards as suggested above.

No Meat

This can be quite controversial for the niche Paleo followers as most of them are vegan or vegetarian. Yes, vegetarian forms of Paleo exist, but you often need to take supplements to keep yourself healthy. It is a universally acknowledged truth that our ancestors devoured meat and we would not have evolved or even survived if they had not. So, drop off your inhibitions and eat meat. Meat is not harmful for your body if consumed in proper form, so drop off salami, bologna, hot dogs etc. from your shopping list and instead add the meats such as elk, grass fed meat etc. As recommended in the Shopping List section of the book, add a lot of seafood to your diet.

Excessive Meat

It is a common misconception that Paleo diet is a meat only diet. Paleo is certainly a meat rich diet but it is nowhere a meat only plan. Paleo diet is based on the diet of our ancestors who were omnivores and not carnivores. It is necessary to eat good amounts of veggies and fruits every day to avoid harmful effects. It is okay and rather necessary to eat meat at least once a day but do not overdo it. If you are trying to lose weight it is better to stick to lean meat, poultry and fish. Too much meat can not only interrupt your weight loss plan but can also cause cardiac and hepatic problems.

Excessive Fruits

Fruits are healthy, notorious and tasty and therefore almost everyone who goes on a diet replaces junk food with fruits. This is a natural and good practice; however, it can take the wrong turn fast. Fruits contain high amounts of fructose- a natural sugar that in high amount can produce excess insulin, which in turn can lead to excess fat storage. So instead of eating a large amount of fruits eat them in moderation and appropriate proportion. You can also replace fruits with cucumbers, celery etc.

Excessive Nuts

Like meat and fruits, it is easy to consume excessive nuts while on the diet. In fact, nuts are perhaps the most overeaten food item, considering their size and taste. Although nuts are allowed and recommended for a good Paleo plan, it is essential to eat them moderation. Do not avoid them as many of them contain Omega 3 and Omega 6. Remember, peanuts are NOT nuts and are NOT Paleo food.

Insufficient Vegetable intake

It is easy to over eat meat and fruits but not vegetables, and hence it is often observed that beginners do not consume enough vegetables. A good Paleo meal should consist of large amount of vegetables to keep you fresh and satiated for a long while supplying you with essential nutrients. Try to pick up vegetables that can be eaten raw in the form of salads, this will reduce your cooking time and you will eat fresh vegetables every time.

Vegetables are also a rich source of fiber that will help you prevent bloating and constipation. However, do not eat potatoes, sweet potatoes, peas etc. in large quantities if you are trying to lose weight. These vegetables are rich sources of starch i.e. carbs. Overeating them will result into weight gain instead of weight loss. You can replace them with cucumbers and other such foods. Instead of eating the above vegetables try to eat lots of spinach, kale, cilantro etc. These are nutrient rich and low calorie vegetables that will help you with your diet.

Spinach also contains a lot of calcium and thus holds an important position in the Paleo world. As Paleo is often a dairy free diet you might not get enough calcium every day. However, if you eat spinach everyday your daily requirements will be met without using any supplements.

Wrong Condiments and Oils

We have seen how simple food items like soy sauce can throw off your diet. Similarly, your cooking oil can cause problems as well. A considerable number of people around the world use corn oil, canola oil or soybean oil all of which are bad for Paleo. Instead, try replacing them with Paleo friendly oils such olive oil, coconut oil etc. Lard can be used as well. Oils such as avocado oil, walnut oil, and almond oil can be used for cold applications. Do not hesitate to include a moderate portion of fats in your diet. However, avoid overdoing it if you are trying to lose weight.

Not Keeping a List of Things Allowed and Things Not Allowed

Although the Paleo diet is a considerably free diet there are still many things that are not Paleo friendly. A simple mistake will set off a time bomb that will destroy your diet routine. Always keep an eye on the lists of "Not Allowed" items. If you are not sure about a food item, just run it once through the list just to be sure. You will find an extensive To Avoid list at the end of this chapter that you can paste around your workspace or carry around with you. If you find carrying papers cumbersome you can also download various apps that are available on app stores.

Choosing the Wrong Paleo

This is one of the most common mistakes people make regarding Paleo diet. There are many versions of Paleo diet that cater to different needs. If you choose to take up an athletic diet to lose weight, you might end up gaining some instead. This is because Paleo is not necessarily a carb-free diet. It has carbs. Food items such as sweet potatoes and bananas are carb rich food items. So, if you are trying to lose weight it is necessary to go on a low carb Paleo diet.

A good low carb Paleo diet will contain high amounts of proteins, moderate amounts of fats and moderate or just the required amounts of carbs. This means avoid bananas and potatoes etc. as much a possible but do not throw them away. You can eat them occasionally.

There are several Paleo diet options available for you. In a few weeks of following this diet, if you do not notice any change, simply stop and start afresh with a new diet plan.

Wrong Portion Sizes

Yes, we said that you could eat all that you want on a Paleo diet. However, if you want to lose weight it is necessary to control your portions. You can eat large portions of vegetables; however, it is necessary to avoid eating too many servings of nuts, avocado, oil, fruits etc. This is also true regarding Paleo deserts. Thanks to various ingenious cooks all around, you can find a Paleo version of almost every dish possible, so you can have Paleo cookies, Paleo cakes, Paleo muffins etc. Now though Paleo versions of these items are considerably healthier than their normal counterparts they still pack a lot of calories that will prevent weight loss. It is necessary to moderate these 'treats'. Instead pick up fruits etc. as desserts.

Eating less is a Paleo sin too! Do not avoid food and ignore hunger. Understand the difference between hunger and cravings. Eat enough to feel satiated. Remember, Paleo is not a starving diet unlike others, so eat healthy and wholesome meals.

Eating Only Certain Kinds of Meat

Everyone loves bacon, but like we mentioned earlier, you have to have variety in your diet. Focus on eating leaner meats, as they are low in calorie. Eating only bacon or any other form of meat will ruin your diet and will slow down weight loss.

Consuming Alcohol

One of the most popular forms of alcohol is beer, which is made of grains. It is better to avoid alcohol on Paleo diet however if you do want to indulge only drink/use gluten free alcohols. Treat alcohol as treats and drink it sparingly.

Overloading Protein

If you eat protein rich food all the time without adding a healthy amount of fats to the diet, not only will you feel constantly hungry but also it will cause fatigue. Add good amount of wholesome, Paleo friendly fats such as coconut oil to your diet.

Excessive Perfection

As said numerous times already, Paleo diet is not a fad diet. It is a lifestyle choice that results into permanent changes. Although it is always recommended to adhere strictly to your meal plan you will realize that it is an exhausting process. Hence, do not punish yourself if you slip for a day or two while on your plan and do not let it ruin your whole diet. Start afresh the next day. Constant denial and deprival is stressful and should be avoided.

But this doesn't mean you should succumb to your cravings all the time.

Obsessing Over Ingredient Quality

A lot of beginners who are new to Paleo often commit the most amateur mistake, obsessing over the quality of the ingredients. Yes, grass fed meat and organic vegetables are better than supermarket meat and veggies but they are also very costly. If you plan to go on a Paleo diet while being on a tight budget your grocery budget will hit the skies if you force on buying organic produces.

Remember, Paleo is for everyone and if someone tells you that you should not be eating grain fed meat, ignore. Buy grass fed meat whenever you can afford it else stick to grain fed meat. Buy the best quality food that you can afford while avoiding non-Paleo items however always read labels. Do not buy any product that has a lot of chemicals on the label, it is non-Paleo.

For people who want to do Paleo diet on a tight budget it is recommended to avoid buying a lot of Paleo baking ingredients. These are often quite costly and you shouldn't be eating them a lot either.

Trusting labels

As mentioned in the last point nowadays it has become quite easy to find products labeled as Paleo or Paleo friendly. Do not trust these products on this label alone. There exists no specific

Paleo regulations board and hence these products cannot be trusted until you read the ingredients carefully. Often Paleo labeled bars and snacks contain high amounts of sugar and chemicals that make them non-Paleo. Scrutinize labels carefully and avoid anything that contains artificial sugar.

The Gluten Dilemma

Although it is highly recommended to avoid gluten rich processed food, it is not recommended to replace it with gluten free processed food. You won't reap many benefits from the latter as it is almost the same as the prior.

Avoiding Sunlight

Remember our ancestors got ample sunlight which supplied them with essential nutrient like Vitamin D. Likewise while following Paleo it is necessary to bask in early morning sun to get enough vitamin D that cannot be procured from diet. If you go for walks, do it early morning so that you can kill two birds with one stone.

Not Using Technology

Yes, Paleo diet is also known as caveman diet. However, that does not mean that you must adopt the lifestyle of the cavemen. Use technology and download Paleo apps that will make your Paleo journey incredibly easy. You can find apps for almost all major OS platforms including IOs, Android, and Windows etc.

These were some of the most common mistakes that should be avoided while following a Paleo diet for weight loss, now as promised let us have a look at an extensive list of what to avoid while following a Paleo diet.

Foods to Avoid

All Forms of Dairy including:

- Whole Milk *

- Yogurt

- Skim Milk

- Low Fat Milk

- Cheese

- Cream Cheese

- Butter *

- Not-fat creamer

- Powdered Milk

- Cottage Cheese

- Ice Milk

- Pudding

- Dairy Spreads

- Fro-Yo

- 2% Milk

- Ice Cream

If you find Paleo recipes that call for milk or milk related products, just replace them with almond milk and milk products.

Beverages

- Coca Cola

- Pepsi

- Sprite

- Mountain Dew

- Red Bull

- Other Sodas and Energy Drinks

- Beer

- Wine

- Other Alcoholic Beverages *

- Apple Juice *

- Grape Juice *

- Orange Juice *

- Mango Juice *

- Strawberry Juice *

- Starfruit Juice *

- Pineapple Juice *

- Coffee *

- Tea *

Grains and Related Products

- Rice

- Wheat

- Barley

- Oats

- Corn

- Soybean

- Breads

- Cereals

- Crackers

- Corn syrup

- Pasta

- Hash browns

- Cream of Wheat

- Oatmeal

Legumes

- All Beans Including
  - Broad beans
  - Black beans
  - Kidney beans
  - Fava beans
  - Horse beans
  - Garbanzo beans
  - Mung beans
  - Pinto beans
  - Lima beans
  - Navy beans
  - Green beans
  - Adzuki beans
  - Red beans
  - String beans
  - White beans

Peas

All Dried Peas including

- Black eyed peas

- Snow peas

- Chickpeas

- Sugar snap peas

Peanuts and Peanut Products like Peanut Butter

- Lentils

- Miso

- Mesquite

- Lupins

- Tofu

- Soymilk

Artificial Sweeteners

- Isomalt

- Sugar Alcohol

- Decomalt

- ClearCut Isomalt

- Isomaltitol

- Hydrogenated Isomatulose
- DiabetiSwee
- Aspartame
- APM
- Equal Classic
- Aspartyl-phenylalanie-1methyl ester
- NutraSweet
- NatraTaste Blue
- Erythritol
- Glycerol
- Glycyrrhizin
- Saccharin
- HSH or Hydrogenated Starch Hydrolysate
- Lactitol
- Maltitol
- Acesulfame Potassium
- Mannitol
- Neotame Xylitol
- Polydextrose

- Sucralose

- Sorbitol

- Steviol glycoside

- Tagatose

Meat

- Spam

- Low Quality Meat

- Hot Dogs

- Highly Processed Supermarket Meat

Snacks

- Ketchup

- French Fries

- Chips

- Pretzels

- Cookies

- Pizza

Vegetables *

- Potatoes

- Acorn Squash

- Yam
- Sweet Potatoes
- Yucca
- Beets
- Butternut Squash

Sweets

- Candy bar
- Chocolate Bars
- 100 Grand
- Milky way
- Hershey's
- Red Vines
- Reese's
- M&Ms
- Snickers
- Twix
- Muffins
- Cakes
- Pastries

Products marked with a '' sign are allowed on some Paleo diets, however consume in moderation.

Chapter 6: FAQs or Frequently Asked Questions

Till now we have seen chapters regarding basics of Paleo diet, how to do a Paleo diet and the common mistakes associated with Paleo diet. However, a lot of you still must have questions and queries in your minds regarding Paleo. Hence, in this chapter we will try to solve some of the most frequently asked questions about Paleo.

What is Paleo?

We have covered this question quite extensively in the first chapter of this book. What foods should I eat? /What foods are not Paleo? Is (insert name) Paleo?

You can find a list of things that are Paleo and non-Paleo in the above chapters. Stick to the list as much as possible. If you cannot find a specific item on the list, a simple Internet search will help you find anything you want. You can also download various Paleo food lists app.

Is Paleo suitable for me?

If you are okay with idea of removing two food groups from your diet and are sure that you can control your body and mind, then yes Paleo is right for you. With this if you are okay with meat and meat products and trust the science behind Paleo diet, you can surely go ahead on the Paleo path.

What makes Paleo Diet Different than Others?

Paleo diet is situated in evolution and is science backed. Unlike fad diets Paleo does not promise to serve as a quick weight loss method rather it promises to be a holistic approach towards weight loss and a healthy lifestyle.

Does it Really Work?

Yes. Paleo diet does work, however do not fall prey to tall and untrue claims. You cannot eat tons of food on Paleo and still lose weight. It will work only when you understand the concept of moderate portions. This is a long-term process and not a quick weight loss method.

I don't know what to cook, are there any recipes available?

Yes. The Internet is full of very innovative Paleo friendly recipes. You can find recipe for almost anything you want to eat including Paleo muffins, Paleo lasagna, Paleo cakes etc.

How do I begin?

You can find a detailed chapter answering this question in this book. Refer to chapter 1.

Is Paleo gluten free?

Yes, Paleo is gluten free, as it is basically grain free. But not all gluten free diets are Paleo as many diets include dairy, legumes etc. that are free of gluten but are not Paleo friendly.

Will I have enough energy?

Yes. The mechanism of our body is such that it can easily survive on a low carb diet. However, if you are an athlete or engage in various physical labors it is advised to modify your diet accordingly.

Is Paleo diet a no-carb diet or a low-carb diet? Are all carbs inherently bad?

Paleo is basically a low-carb diet that you can modify per your requirements. No carbs are inherently bad, and they do have a purpose in our diet. Carbs are important energy sources and as stated above Paleo diet does include various carbs sources. However, instead of focusing on carb-laden foods like grains, Paleo diet allows you to get your carbs from more natural sources like vegetables and fruits.

Is dairy Paleo friendly?

The answer is Yes and No. No animal willingly drinks milk after infancy except humans. Hence, it is safe to assume that cavemen did not drink milk, at least not regularly hence a lot of followers tend to avoid diary. However, if you like dairy and are not lactose intolerant you can consume it sparingly. People who are trying to lose weight should avoid it altogether.

I have heard Paleo is a fat rich diet, isn't fat bad for you?

No, Paleo is not inherently bad. In fact, if you want to follow a regular Paleo diet successfully fats are essential. Carbs are our largest source of energy and as Paleo diet is all about cutting off carbs you might be left without any energy at all. This need is then fulfilled by fats. So, consume a healthy amount of fats everyday while on Paleo. However, if you are trying to lose weight do not consume excessive fats.

When do I eat? How many times should I eat?

There is no fixed eating schedule in Paleo. You are free to eat whenever you feel hungry. On the other hand, you can afford to go without food all day long if you don't feel hungry. You don't have to eat every three hours like many other diets. You can easily skip meals if you feel like; but at the same time do not curb your hunger. If you do happen to skip meals, do not overeat at a later time. If you are an athlete eat, then it's vital to eat frequently.

Is Paleo low calorie/ low glycemic diet?

Paleo is not inherently a low-calorie diet however it contains fewer calories that of an average American diet. Paleo isn't inherently a low glycemic diet either; but it can be made low glycemic by consulting a nutritionist.

Is Paleo easy?

Difficulty is a subjective concept, what is difficult for individual will be a piece of cake for other. Hence, you can try out the diet for a month and decide for yourself. If you feel that the diet is too difficult for you, modify the diet plan accordingly.

Is Paleo a protein rich diet and can I used it to build muscles?

Yes, Paleo is a protein rich diet thanks to the amount of meat that is consumed. You can add weight training to your routine while following a Paleo diet; however do consult your nutritionist before starting a new regime.

Can I consume sugar while on Paleo?

Yes and No again. Natural sugar such as maple syrup, honey, fruits etc. are allowed on Paleo, everything else including refined sugar isn't.

Is Paleo safe for pregnant women?

Yes, Paleo is safe for pregnant women. However, it is highly recommended to consult your Ob-Gyn before starting any new diet while being pregnant.

Is Paleo vegan?

No. Paleo is not vegan. You may find certain versions of Paleo that claim to be vegan, however most of them make you eat a variety of chemicals and supplements.

Does Paleo cause acne?

There is no valid proof of Paleo causing acne. However, if you are prone to acne you might break out in the first few weeks of Paleo, as your body will go through a transition.

Does Paleo cause constipation?

If you eat enough veggies along with plentiful of water every day you won't be constipated. However, if you are prone to constipation add a spoonful or two of flaxseed to your diet every day.

Will I lose my hair?

No, Paleo does not result into hair loss. However, you might notice some hair fall in the first week of Paleo, as your body will go through transition.

Conclusion

Thank you for choosing this book and we hope that you enjoyed it. The goal of this book was to inform you about the basics of Paleo diet and to make you aware of the common mistakes that many beginners commit. We sincerely hope that we achieved the goal.

All the advice given in this book is tried and tested and thus is sure to work. You can start the diet immediately without any inhibition. You can start instantly by following our basic diet guidelines chapter.

It is recommended to stay on this diet for at least a month to reap its benefits. It is also recommended to pick up a few Paleo friendly recipe books that will help you on your Paleo diet routine.

Good Luck!